KNOW MORE ABOUT YOUR LIVER

The greatest guide to diagnosing, treating, and preventing all liver diseases.

by

Kenneth B. Wright

TABLE OF CONTENTS

Know more about your liver

Know more about your liver

INTRODUCTION

According to the American Liver Foundation, roughly thirty million persons in the United States have been diagnosed with liver disease. That means one out of every 10 persons is affected by a disease such as hepatitis, cirrhosis, or liver cancer. Even though your liver is critical to sustaining a healthy existence since it performs several important processes in the body, it is often disregarded. The alarming element about liver illness is that you can have one for a long period without being aware that something is wrong. It is only when the problem has substantially worsened that you begin to experience its symptoms and grasp the effect it might have on your health. That is why it is so crucial to know about the risk factors and earliest indicators of liver illnesses. The earlier you can catch a liver disease, the better your prognosis will be. *Know more about your liver* will give you the key information you need to know to gain insight into how well your liver is performing. You will be able to discover your risk factors for liver disease, as well as the critical steps you can take to avoid one from happening in the first place. if you have already been diagnosed with a liver illness, it is crucial to understand your treatment and management choices, which will also be explored in this book.

The purpose of this book is to provide you with the essentials of liver disease. Because liver illness can be complex, understanding the essentials is crucial for you to effectively engage with your doctor and other healthcare providers in establishing a treatment plan.

This is supposed to be a beginner-level book that gives you the information you need in a simple read-and-understand format.

Through reading this book, you will get knowledge not just of the dietary and lifestyle modifications that you can make to improve your liver health, but also of the clinical side of various illnesses so that you may effectively work with your health care provider to build a personalized treatment.

Whether you have the risk factors for liver disease (but have not been diagnosed with one) or you have been living with a liver illness for years, this book empowers you with the tools and information that you need to give yourself the best possible outcome. The knowledge that you receive from this book will allow you to be your champion for your health care. Let's get reading!

Chapter 1

THE LIVER

The liver is the largest solid organ found in the human body. It eliminates pollutants from the body's blood supply, maintains healthy blood sugar levels, controls blood clotting, and conducts hundreds of other critical activities. It is placed beneath the rib cage in the right upper abdomen.

Key Facts about the liver

- The liver filters all of the blood in the body and breaks down toxic chemicals, such as alcohol and narcotics.
- The liver also generates bile, a fluid that helps digest fats and carries away waste.
- The liver consists of four lobes, which are each made up of eight sections and thousands of lobules (or small lobes).

Functions of the Liver

The liver is an essential organ of the body that performs over 500 crucial activities.

These include eliminating waste items and foreign substances from the bloodstream, regulating blood sugar levels and producing necessary nutrients.

Below are some of its most crucial functions:

Albumin Production: Albumin is a protein that stops fluids in the bloodstream from seeping into surrounding tissue. It also delivers hormones, vitamins, and enzymes through the body.

Bile Production: Bile is a fluid that is crucial to the digestion and absorption of lipids in the small intestine.

Filters Blood: All the blood exiting the stomach and intestines travels via the liver, which eliminates toxins, byproducts, and other dangerous compounds.

Regulates Amino Acids: The creation of proteins depend on amino acids. The liver makes sure amino acid levels in the bloodstream stay healthy.

Regulates Blood Clotting: Blood clotting coagulants are formed utilizing vitamin K, which can only be absorbed with the help of bile, a fluid th liver generates.

Resists Infections: As part of the filtering process, the liver also eliminates microorganisms from the bloodstream.

Stores Vitamins and Minerals: The liver stores considerable amounts of vitamins A, D, E, K, and B12, as well as iron and copper.

Processes Glucose: The liver eliminates excess glucose (sugar) from the bloodstream and stores it as glycogen. As needed, it can transform glycogen back into glucose.

Anatomy of the Liver

The liver is reddish-brown and formed essentially like a cone or a wedge, with the tiny end above the spleen and stomach and the large end above the small intestine. The entire organ is placed below the lungs in the right upper abdomen. It weights between 3 and 3.5 pounds.

Structure of the liver

The liver comprises of four lobes: the bigger right lobe and left lobe, and the smaller caudate lobe and quadrate lobe. The left and right lobe are split by the falciform ("sickle-shaped" in Latin) ligament, which joins the liver to the abdominal wall. The liver's lobes can be further split into eight segments, which are made up of thousands of lobules (little lobes). Each of these lobules has a duct going toward the common hepatic duct, which drains bile from the liver.

Parts of the liver

The following are some of the most essential individual sections of the liver:

Common Hepatic Duct: A tube that transports bile out of the liver. It is created from the intersection of the right and left hepatic ducts.

Falciform Ligament: A thin, fibrous ligament that divides the two lobes of the liver and attaches it to the abdominal wall.

Glisson's Capsule: A layer of loose connective tissue that surrounds the liver and its accompanying arteries and ducts.

Hepatic Artery: The major blood vessel which supplies the liver with oxygenated blood.

Hepatic Portal Vein: The blood vessel which carries blood from the gastrointestinal tract, gallbladder, pancreas, and spleen to the liver.

Lobes: The anatomical sections of the liver.

Lobules: Microscopic building blocks of the liver.

Peritoneum: A membrane which covers the liver that forms the exterior.

Maintaining a Healthy Liver

The greatest method to avoid liver disease is to take active measures toward a healthy life. The following are some guidelines that will assist keep the liver operating as it should:

1. **Avoid Illicit Drugs:** Illicit drugs are toxins that the liver must filter out. Taking these medicines can create long-term damage.
2. **Drink Alcohol Moderately:** Alcohol must be broken down by the liver. While the liver can modulate levels, excessive alcohol usage can cause damage.
3. **Exercise Regularly:** A regular exercise plan will help enhance general health for every organ, including the liver.
4. **Eat Healthy Foods:** Eating excessive fats can make it difficult for the liver to function and lead to fatty liver disease.
5. **Practice Safe Sex:** Use protection to avoid sexually transmitted diseases such as hepatitis C.
6. **Vaccinate:** Especially before traveling, receive proper vaccines against hepatitis A and B, as well as

diseases such as malaria and yellow fever, which thrive in the liver.

Liver Disease

There are several types of liver illness. Some of the more common forms are curable with diet and lifestyle modifications, while others may require lifetime medication to maintain.

If you begin treatment early enough, you can often avert lasting damage. There might be no symptoms in the early stages. Late-stage liver disease is more difficult to treat.

Your liver is a huge and powerful organ that conducts hundreds of critical processes in your body. One of its most significant duties is filtering poisons from your blood. While your liver is well-equipped for this duty, its role as a filter renders it sensitive to the toxins it processes. Too many pollutants might overload your liver's resources and capacity to function. This might happen temporarily or over a lengthy period of time.

When healthcare providers refer to liver disease, they're usually talking to chronic illnesses that produce progressive harm to your liver over time.

Viral infections, toxic poisoning and certain metabolic disorders are among the primary causes of chronic liver disease. Your liver has remarkable healing powers, but constantly working overtime to restore itself takes its toll. Eventually, it can't keep up.

What are the stages of chronic liver disease?
Chronic liver disease progresses in about four stages:

- Hepatitis.

- Fibrosis.

- Cirrhosis.

- Liver failure

Chapter 2

Hepatitis

Hepatitis is an inflammation of the liver. It may be caused by viral infection, alcohol consumption, many health issues, or even some drugs. Treatment varies depends on the nature and underlying reason.

Hepatitis is an inflammatory disorder of the liver. It is often the result of a viral infection; however there are other probable causes of hepatitis.

These include autoimmune hepatitis and hepatitis that occurs as a secondary effect of medications, narcotics, poisons, and alcohol. Autoimmune hepatitis is a disease that arises when your body creates antibodies against your liver tissue.

The five basic viral classifications of hepatitis are hepatitis A, B, C, D, and E. A separate virus is responsible for each kind of viral hepatitis.

The World Health Organization (WHO) estimates that 354 million people currently live with chronic hepatitis B and C globally.

Hepatitis A

Hepatitis A is the outcome of an infection with the hepatitis A virus (HAV). This kind of hepatitis is an acute, short-term condition.

Hepatitis B

The hepatitis B virus (HBV) causes hepatitis B. This is generally a persistent, chronic problem. The Centers for Disease Control and Prevention (CDC) estimates that over 826,000 persons are living with chronic hepatitis B in the United States and around 257 million people globally.

Hepatitis C

Hepatitis C comes from the hepatitis C virus (HCV). HCV is among the most frequent blood borne viral infections in the United States and often appears as a long-term disease.

According to the CDC, approximately 2.4 million Americans are now living with a chronic version of this condition.

Hepatitis D

This is an uncommon form of hepatitis that exclusively arises in association with hepatitis B infection. The hepatitis D virus (HDV) produces liver inflammation like other strains; however a person cannot get HDV without an existing hepatitis B infection.

Globally, HDV affects almost 5 patients with chronic hepatitis B.

Hepatitis E

Hepatitis E is a waterborne disease that occurs from exposure to the hepatitis E virus (HEV). Hepatitis E is mainly common in places with inadequate sanitation and typically results from swallowing fecal matter that contaminates the water supply.

This disease is uncommon in the United States, according to the CDC.

Hepatitis E is usually acute but can be extremely hazardous in pregnant women.

Causes of hepatitis

Hepatitis A can be caused by exposure to HAV in food or water.

Hepatitis B is caused by contact with HBV in body fluids, such as blood, vaginal secretions, or semen

Hepatitis C is caused by contact with HCV in body fluids, such as blood, vaginal secretions, or semen.

Hepatitis D is majorly caused by contact with blood harboring HDV.

Hepatitis E emanates from exposure to HEV in food or drink.

Causes of noninfectious hepatitis

Although hepatitis is most usually the outcome of an infection, other reasons can cause the illness.

Alcohol and other poisons

Excess alcohol intake can cause liver damage and inflammation. This may also be called alcoholic hepatitis.

The alcohol immediately injures the cells of your liver. Over time, it can cause irreversible damage and lead to thickening or scarring of liver tissue (cirrhosis) and liver failure.

Other hazardous causes of hepatitis include abuse of drugs and exposure to chemicals.

Autoimmune system reaction
In rare situations, the immune system interprets the liver as toxic and attacks it. This creates chronic inflammation that can range from mild to severe, typically impairing liver function. It's three times more common in women than in males.

Common symptoms of hepatitis

If you are living with a chronic form of hepatitis, including hepatitis B and C, you may not display symptoms until the damage compromises liver function. By contrast, persons with acute hepatitis may show with symptoms immediately after receiving a hepatitis virus.
Common signs of infectious hepatitis include:

- fatigue
- flu-like symptoms
- dark urine
- pale stool
- abdominal pain

- loss of appetite
- unexpected weight loss

- yellow skin and eyes, which may be indicators of jaundice

How hepatitis is diagnosed

It is vital to understand what is causing hepatitis in order to treat it effectively. Doctors will progress through a battery of tests to accurately identify your problem.

To diagnose all forms of hepatitis, your doctor will first check your history to discover any risk factors you may have.

During a physical examination, your doctor may press down gently on your abdomen to discover whether there's pain or soreness. Your doctor may also check for any swelling of the liver and any yellow coloring in your eyes or skin.

Liver function tests

Liver function tests use blood samples to measure how efficiently your liver works.

Abnormal findings of these tests may be the first clue that there is a problem, especially if you don't show any indicators on a physical exam of liver disease. High liver enzyme levels may indicate that your liver is strained, damaged, or not functioning adequately.

Other blood tests

If your liver function tests are abnormal, your doctor will likely prescribe more blood tests to discover the source of the problem.

These tests can determine if you have infectious hepatitis by looking for the presence of hepatitis viruses or antibodies your body makes to battle them.

Doctors may also use blood tests to check for any evidence of autoimmune hepatitis.

Liver biopsy

When diagnosing hepatitis, doctors will also check your liver for potential damage.

A liver biopsy is a technique that includes obtaining a sample of tissue from your liver.

A medical expert may take this sample via your skin with a needle, meaning there is no need for surgery. They will often use an ultrasound scan for guidance throughout this treatment.

This test allows your doctor to detect how infection or inflammation has impacted your liver.

Ultrasound

An abdominal ultrasound uses ultrasound waves to create an image of the organs within your belly. This test lets your doctor to take a close look at your liver and adjacent organs. It can reveal:

Fluid in your abdomen

Liver damage or hypertrophy

Liver tumors

Anomalies of your gallbladder
Sometimes the pancreas shows up on ultrasound pictures as well.

This can be a beneficial test in establishing the source of your abnormal liver function.

How hepatitis is treated
Treatment choices will differ on the type of hepatitis you have and whether the infection is acute or persistent.

Hepatitis A
Hepatitis A is a short-term infection and may not require treatment. However, if symptoms cause a large degree of discomfort, bed rest may be necessary. In

addition, if you experience vomiting or diarrhea, your doctor may recommend a nutritional program to maintain your hydration and nutrients.

Hepatitis B

There is no specific treatment approach for acute hepatitis B.

However, if you have chronic hepatitis B, you will require antiviral medicines. This sort of treatment can be pricey, as you may have to continue it for several months or years.

Treatment for chronic hepatitis B also requires regular medical evaluations and monitoring to evaluate if the virus is responding to treatment.

Hepatitis C

Antiviral medicines can treat both acute and chronic forms of hepatitis C.

Typically, persons who develop chronic hepatitis C will require a combination of antiviral medication regimens. They may also need more tests to establish the best method of treatment.

People who develop cirrhosis or liver damage owing to chronic hepatitis C may be candidates for a liver transplant.

Hepatitis D

The World health organization (WHO) lists pegylated interferon alpha as a therapy for hepatitis D. However, this medicine can have serious negative effects. As a result, it's not recommended for those with cirrhosis liver damage, those with psychological disorders, and people with autoimmune diseases.

Hepatitis E

Currently, no specific medical therapies are available to treat Hepatitis E because the infection is often acute, it typically resolves on its own.

Doctors would often urge persons with this infection to get appropriate rest, drink plenty of fluids, acquire enough nutrients, and avoid alcohol. However, pregnant women who get this illness require special monitoring and treatment.

Autoimmune hepatitis

Corticosteroids, such prednisone or budesonide, are highly crucial in the early therapy of autoimmune hepatitis. They're successful in about 80 percent of persons with this illness.

Azathioprine (Imuran), a medication that inhibits the immune system, may also be a part of therapy programs. This can be used with or without steroids.

Other immune-suppressing medications such mycophenolate (CellCept), tacrolimus (Prograf), and cyclosporine (Neoral) can also be used instead of azathioprine in treatment

Tips to prevent hepatitis

There are vaccinations that can help protect against several hepatitis viruses. Minimizing your risk of exposure to drugs containing these viruses can also be an effective preventive approach.

Vaccines

A vaccine for hepatitis A can help prevent the contraction of HAV. The hepatitis A vaccine is a series of double doses and most children begin vaccination at age 12 to 23 months. This is also available for adults and can include the hepatitis B vaccine.

The CDC recommends hepatitis B vaccines for all babies. Doctors commonly deliver the sequence of three immunizations over the first 6 months of childhood.

The CDC also recommends the immunization for all healthcare and medical staff. Vaccination against hepatitis B may assist in preventing hepatitis D.

There are presently no vaccinations for hepatitis C or E.

Reducing exposure

Hepatitis viruses can pass from person to person by contact with bodily fluids, water, and foods harboring infectious agents. Minimizing your risk of contact with these substances can assist to prevent developing hepatitis viruses.

Practicing excellent hygiene is one strategy to avoid catching hepatitis A and E. The viruses that cause these conditions are present in water. If you're traveling to a place where there is a high prevalence of hepatitis, you should avoid, local water, ice, uncooked or undercooked seafood and oysters, raw fruit and veggies.

The hepatitis B, C, and D viruses can transfer by contact with bodily fluids carrying these infectious agents. You can reduce your risk of coming into contact with fluids carrying these viruses by:

- Not sharing needles
- Not sharing razors
- Not using someone else's toothbrush
- Not touching spilled blood

Hepatitis B and C can come through sexual intercourse and sexual contact. Using barrier techniques, such as condoms and dental dams, during sexual activity can help lower the risk of infection.

Complications of hepatitis

Chronic hepatitis B or C can lead to more severe health concerns. Because the virus affects the liver, patients with chronic hepatitis B or C are at risk of:

- Chronic liver disease.
- Cirrhosis.
- Liver cancer.

When your liver stops functioning normally, liver failure can result. Complications of liver failure include:

- Bleeding disorders.
- A collection of fluid in your abdomen, known as ascites.
- Elevated blood pressure in portal veins that enter your liver, known as portal hypertension.
- Renal failure.

- Hepatic encephalopathy, which can cause weariness, memory loss, and reduced mental ability
- Hepatocellular carcinoma, which is a sort of liver cancer
- Death

People with chronic hepatitis B and C should avoid alcohol as it can accelerate liver damage and failure. Certain vitamins and drugs might also impact liver function. If you have chronic hepatitis B or C, check with your doctor before taking any new drugs

Chapter 3

Fibrosis

Fibrosis is a slow hardening of your liver as thin bands of scar tissue gradually add up. Scar tissue limits blood flow through your liver, which reduces its availability to oxygen and nutrients. This is how your liver's vitality begins to progressively deteriorate. Remarkably, some amount of fibrosis is reversible. Your liver cells can renew, and scarring can lessen if the damage slows down sufficiently for it to heal.

Liver fibrosis happens when the healthy tissue of your liver gets scarred and cannot perform as well. Fibrosis is the first level of liver scarring. Some fibrosis can be reversible.

Scarring of the liver occurs on a spectrum, with variable degrees. Some of them may be treated and reversible. However, drugs and lifestyle modifications can help to keep fibrosis from getting worse.

There are various distinct scales of liver fibrosis staging, where a specialist determines the degree of liver damage. This may be performed with a variety of procedures, including as blood testing, imaging tests, and a tissue biopsy that may be further studied under a microscope (histology).

But first, a doctor will need to diagnose any underlying chronic liver illness, such as fatty liver disease or hepatitis. This can assist uncover the underlying causes of inflammation that lead to fibrosis, and better guide the staging and therapy process.

While fibrosis staging can assist you and a doctor understand the degree to which your liver can be affected, it's crucial to emphasize that the pinpointing the underlying reason is more important than focusing on any one stage.

If a liver biopsy and histology is performed, a clinician may stage liver fibrosis based on the METAVIR grading system.

This assigns a "score" which depends on two factors: inflammation (activity) and damage (fibrosis). A lower number may indicate less inflammation and damage, whereas a higher score could mean more.

The activity grades range from A0 to A3:

A0: no activity

A1: modest activity

A2: moderate activity

A3: extreme activity

The fibrosis phases range from F0 to F4:

F0: no fibrosis

F1: portal fibrosis without septa

F2: portal fibrosis with little septa

F3: many septa without cirrhosis

F4: cirrhosis

Therefore, a person with the most severe disease form may have an A3, F4 METAVIR score.

Another rating method based in histology is Batts and Ludwig, which grades fibrosis on a scale of grade 1 to grade 4, with grade 4 being the most severe.
The International Association of the Study of the Liver (IASL) also offers a histological scoring system with four categories that include:

- Minimal chronic hepatitis

- Mild chronic hepatitis

- Moderate chronic hepatitis

- Severe chronic hepatitis

Fibrosis staging may also be dependent on other tests outside of a liver biopsy and histology. For example, a clinician may confirm liver fibrosis with a blood test that detects fibrosis 4 (Fib4) in the blood.
A score of less than 1.3 may be deemed low-risk, while a Fib4 level of more than 3.25 could imply you're at a high risk for liver fibrosis.

Additionally, fibrosis staging may be established with the use of imaging examinations. These look at the size and form of you liver, as well as for extra fat, tumors, or shrinking. Possible imaging study techniques include:

1. Abdominal ultrasound

2. Computed tomography (CT) scan of your abdomen

3. Magnetic resonance imaging (MRI) scan

4. Elastography, which is paired with either an ultrasound or MRI scan

What are the symptoms of liver fibrosis?

Doctors don't commonly diagnose liver fibrosis in its mild to moderate stages. This is because liver fibrosis doesn't normally show symptoms until more of the liver is affected.

When a person does develop in their liver disease, they may encounter symptoms that include:

- appetite loss

- difficulties thinking clearly

- fluid buildup in the legs or stomach

- jaundice (where the skin and eyes appear yellow)

- nausea

- unexpected weight loss

- weakness

What are the causes of liver fibrosis?

Liver fibrosis occurs after a person encounters injury or inflammation in the liver. The liver's cells stimulate wound healing. During this wound healing, extra proteins such as collagen and glycoproteins build up in the liver.

Eventually, after multiple episodes of repair, the liver cells (known as hepatocytes) can no longer repair themselves. The extra proteins cause scar tissue or fibrosis.

Several forms of liver disorders exist that can cause fibrosis. These include:

- autoimmune hepatitis

- biliary blockage

- iron overload

- viral hepatitis B and C

- alcoholic liver disease

The most prevalent cause of liver fibrosis is nonalcoholic fatty liver disease (NAFLD), whereas the second is alcoholic liver disease due to long-term excesses of consuming alcohol.

Treatment options

Treatment options for liver fibrosis largely rely upon the underlying etiology of the fibrosis. A doctor will treat the underlying ailment, if possible, to decrease the impact of liver disease.

For example, if a person drinks alcohol excessively, a doctor may recommend a treatment program to assist them stop drinking. If a person has NAFLD, a doctor may prescribe adopting dietary adjustments to lose weight and taking drugs to improve better blood sugar management.

Exercising and decreasing weight may also assist to limit the disease's progression.

Treatments for particular causes of liver fibrosis include:

- **chronic liver disease:** ACE inhibitors, which includes benazepril, Lisinopril, and ramipril.

- **hepatitis C virus:** direct action antivirals such as Epclusa, Harvoni, Mayvret, etc.

- **nonalcoholic steatohepatitis:** PPAR-alpha agonist.

- **Autoimmunhepatitis:**immunosuppressive treatment.

- **alcohol liver disease:** abstinence from alcohol

A doctor may also recommend antifibrotics that may possibly help lessen the possibility of irreversible liver scarring (cirrhosis). Depending on the type of drug, antifibrotics are classified as:

anti-inflammatories: examples include belapectin, cenicriviroc, and liraglutide hepatocyte apoptosis inhibitors: these include emricasan, pentoxifylline, and selonsertib oxidative stress inhibitors: options include methyl ferulic acid and losartan.

hepatic stellate cell (HSC) inhibitors: these medications target several cytokines that may activate HSCs and contribute to fibrosis.

Still, there are limitations to antifibrotic treatment. While several of the above drugs are used for other purposes, such as high blood pressure and vascular illnesses, not all are yet approved for the treatment of liver fibrosis. Animal research show promise, but human clinical trials are restricted.

If a person's liver fibrosis gets to where their liver is highly scarred and doesn't work, a person's only final treatment is often to have a liver transplant. However, the waiting list is considerable for these transplant types and not every person is a surgical candidate.

Diagnosis

Liver biopsy

Usually, doctors considered taking a liver biopsy the "gold standard" of testing for liver fibrosis. This is a surgical technique where a doctor would obtain a tissue sample. A professional known as a pathologist will evaluate the tissue for the presence of scarring or fibrosis.

Transient elastography

Another alternative is an imaging test known as transient elastography. This is a test that examines how rigid the liver is. When a person develops liver fibrosis, the damaged cells make the liver stiffer.

This test employs low-frequency sound waves to measure how rigid liver tissue is. However, it's possible to get false positives where the liver tissue may appear stiff, but a biopsy doesn't demonstrate liver scarring.

Nonsurgical tests

However, doctors have been able to use alternative tests that don't require surgery to determine the risk a person may have liver fibrosis.

Examples are matrix metalloproteinase-1 (MMP), and tissue inhibitor of matrix metalloproteinase-1 (TIMP-1). Doctors may also utilize tests that require mathematics, such as an aminotransferase-to-platelet ratio (APRI) or a blood test called Fibro that assesses six different markers of liver function and puts them into an algorithm before awarding a score.

However, a doctor can't usually tell the stage of liver fibrosis simply on these tests.

Ideally, a doctor will discover a person with liver fibrosis at an early stage when the ailment is more curable.

However, because the ailment doesn't normally create symptoms in earlier stages, doctors don't usually discover the condition earlier.

Complications

The most major complication of liver fibrosis might be liver cirrhosis, or extensive scarring that makes the liver so damaged a person will get sick. Usually, this takes a long time to occur, such as over the period of one or two decades.

A person requires their liver to survive since the liver is responsible for filtering dangerous compounds in the blood and doing many other processes that are necessary to the body.

Ultimately, if a person's fibrosis proceeds to cirrhosis and liver failure, they can suffer consequences such as:

- **ascites** (severe buildup of fluid in the abdomen)
- **hepatic encephalopathy** (buildup of waste products that produces confusion)
- **hepatorenal syndrome**
- **portal hypertension**
- **variceal bleeding**

Chapter 4

Cirrhosis

Cirrhosis is extensive, irreversible scarring in your liver. This stage can be describe as a stage where fibrosis is no longer reversible. When your liver no longer has enough healthy cells left to operate with, its tissues can no longer regenerate. But you can still stop the damage at this stage. Cirrhosis will begin to impact your liver function, but your body will seek to compensate for the loss, so you might not notice at first.

Cirrhosis of the liver is late stage liver disease, in which healthy liver tissue has been gradually replaced with scar tissue. Cirrhosis is a result of long-term, chronic hepatitis. Hepatitis is inflammation in your liver, which has numerous causes. When inflammation is going on, your liver tries to repair itself by scarring. But too much scar tissue inhibits your liver from operating normally. The final stage is chronic liver failure.

Are there phases of cirrhosis?

Cirrhosis is a degenerative disorder that worsens as more and more scar tissue forms. In the beginning, your body adjusts to compensate for your diminished liver function, and you might not notice it too much. This is known as compensated cirrhosis. Eventually, though, as your liver function drops further, you will begin to suffer significant symptoms. This is known as decompensated cirrhosis.

How does cirrhosis affect my liver and body?

Scarring in your liver limits the flow of blood and oxygen through your liver tissues. This reduces your liver's capacity to absorb your blood, digest nutrients and filter out pollutants. Cirrhosis impairs your liver's ability to create bile and vital blood proteins. Scar tissue can also compress blood vessels running through your liver, particularly the important portal vein system, leading to a condition called portal hypertension.

How frequent is cirrhosis?

Cirrhosis is relatively prevalent and is a substantial cause of hospitalization and death, especially beyond middle age. That's because it grows gradually over time. In the United States, cirrhosis affects roughly 0.25% of all individuals and about 0.50% of adults between the ages of 45 and 54. Each year, roughly 26,000 deaths in the United States are due to cirrhosis, and these rates are rising. Cirrhosis is a global health concern.

Symptoms and Causes

What are the indications and symptoms of cirrhosis of the liver?

Signs and symptoms of cirrhosis are based on how advanced it is. You could not have symptoms at all early on, or you might just have nonspecific symptoms that resemble many different disorders. Symptoms of cirrhosis become increasingly visible as your liver function diminishes. For example, you might find indicators that bile isn't moving where it needs to go, and instead is overflowing into places it doesn't belong.

What are the early indicators of cirrhosis of the liver?
Early indications and symptoms of cirrhosis may include:

- Nausea or loss of appetite.

- Feeling weak or fatigued (fatigue).

- Feeling generally sick (malaise).

- Upper abdomen pain (especially on the right).

- Visible blood vessels that look like spiders (spider angiomas).

- Redness on the palms of your hands (palmar erythema).

What are indications of progressing cirrhosis?

Recognizable symptoms of cirrhosis come into two categories: symptoms due to deteriorating liver function and symptoms associated to portal hypertension.

Symptoms of stopped bile flow, such jaundice, are classic indicators of deteriorating liver function. Symptoms of portal hypertension imply cirrhosis particularly. It's scar tissue in your liver that compresses your portal vein.

Cirrhosis symptoms connected to decreased liver function include:

- Jaundice (yellow tinge to your skin and eyes).

- Pruritus (itchy skin, but with no visible rash).

- Dark-colored pee and light-colored feces.

- Digestive issues, especially with lipids.

- Small yellow pimples of fat deposits on your skin or eyelids.

- Unexplained weight loss and muscle loss.

- Hepatic encephalopathy (confusion, disorientation, mood disturbances).

- Motor dysfunction (twitching, tremors or lapses in muscle control).

- Disruptions to your menstrual cycle.

- Enlarged male breast tissue and reduced testes in people AMAB.

Cirrhosis symptoms associated to portal hypertension include:

- Swelling in your abdomen (ascites).

- Swelling in your hands, feet, legs and/or face (edema).

- Easy bleeding and bruising (coagulopathy).

- Blood in your vomit or blood in your poop.

- Low urine output (from chronic renal failure).

- Shortness of breath (from chronic respiratory failure).

What causes cirrhosis of the liver?

Cirrhosis is a progressive scarring process that's produced by chronic inflammation in your liver. Any chronic liver illness that produces chronic hepatitis can develop to cirrhosis. The most common causes include:

Alcohol-induced hepatitis: This is a chronic liver damage from chronic excessive alcohol usage. Alcohol may be the most popular cause of liver cirrhosis, but nonalcoholic reasons are also common.

Non-alcohol-related steatohepatitis: This is persistent damage from increased fat buildup in your liver. It's related to metabolic factors such excessive blood lipids, blood sugar and blood pressure.

Less common causes of cirrhosis include:

Autoimmune biliary disease: Certain autoimmune diseases can induce persistent liver inflammation, including autoimmune hepatitis, primary biliary cholangitis and primary sclerosing cholangitis.

Genetic disorders: Certain genetic disorders can cause harmful compounds to build up in your liver and damage it, such as glycogen storage disease, cystic fibrosis and Wilson disease.

Toxic hepatitis: Long-term exposure to some environmental chemicals or usage of certain medications may induce chronic liver damage, including over-the-counter opioids.

Cardiovascular illness: Conditions that cause blood to build up in your liver (congestive heart failure) or that prevent blood from reaching your liver (chronic ischemia) might damage it.

What are the risk factors for this condition?

You can be at higher risk for cirrhosis of the liver if you:

- Are older than 50.

- Have a history of heavy alcohol usage.

- Have a persistent viral hepatitis infection.

- Have metabolic syndrome.

What are the complications of cirrhosis?

- Downstream implications of cirrhosis and portal hypertension include:

- General toxicity, feeling unwell, fatigued and foggy.

- Reduced immunity, healing and recovery.

- Fluid leaking from your veins, creating edema in your body.

- Hormonal imbalances and inadequacies.

- Digestivedifficulties, malabsorption and malnutrition.

- Mild cognitive impairment and motor dysfunction.

Life-threatening consequences of cirrhosis and portal hypertension can include:

1. Gastrointestinal varices and gastrointestinal hemorrhage.

2. Spontaneous bacterial peritonitis.

3. Kidney failure (hepatorenal syndrome).

4. Respiratory failure (hepatopulmonary syndrome).

How is cirrhosis of the liver diagnosed?

A healthcare physician will begin by physically checking you for signs and symptoms of cirrhosis of the liver. They'll ask you about when your symptoms began and whether they've altered over time. They'll also ask questions about your medical history, what drugs, herbs or supplements you take, and your food and lifestyle. They'll seek for indicators that might reveal a history of liver disease or liver injury.

They'll follow up with medical testing to look for evidence of cirrhosis of the liver. Tests may include:

- Blood testing: A panel of liver function tests can identify symptoms of liver disease and liver failure. These measure liver products like liver enzymes, proteins and bilirubin levels in the human blood.

- Blood testing may also identify certain disorders or recognized negative effects, like impaired blood coagulation.

- Imaging testing: Imaging tests like an abdominal ultrasound, or MRI can show the size, shape and texture of your liver. A unique form of imaging test called elastography uses ultrasound or MRI technologies to detect the level of stiffness or fibrosis in your liver.

- Liver biopsy: A liver biopsy is a minor surgery to extract a small tissue sample from your liver to evaluate in a lab. A healthcare provider can take the sample through a hollow needle. While not usually necessary, a liver biopsy can confirm cirrhosis and may help establish the etiology.

Management and Treatment

Cirrhosis causes chronic scarring in your liver, which can't be undone. While your liver has amazing healing powers in general, cirrhosis is a stage of disease when it doesn't have enough healthy cells left to heal itself with. But you may be able to stop cirrhosis from progressing further.

This depends on what's causing it, how treatable the problem is, and how well you respond to the treatment.

Treatment for cirrhosis of the liver includes:
- Managing the cause, if feasible, to slow or limit the damage.
- General diet and lifestyle recommendations to lessen stress on your liver.
- Managing or screening for complications of cirrhosis.
- As a last resort, liver transplantation.

Treating the cause

Medications can cure various forms of liver ailments, with varied levels of efficacy. For example, antivirals can cure chronic hepatitis C but merely reduce (not cure) chronic hepatitis B. Corticosteroids and immunosuppressants can help treat some autoimmune illnesses, but not all. Other drugs can reverse the effects of certain genetic disorders but may only treat the symptoms of others.

If you have toxic or alcohol-related liver disease, eliminating those toxins from your life is the only solution. Some people may require therapy for a substance use disorder to handle this. If you have nonalcohol-related liver disease, controlling metabolic factors like cholesterol, blood sugar and overweight will help relieve it. Some people may need drugs to assist address these factors.

Diet and lifestyle

Even if your liver illness is from other sources, quitting alcohol and medicines that damage your liver will help protect your liver longer. The same is true of metabolic stress variables. Healthcare specialists say that anyone with any form of liver disease should aim to maintain eat healthy meals and obtain a weight that's healthy for you. In addition, certain patients might need dietary supplements to alleviate nutritional deficiencies.

Treating the complications

Once your healthcare practitioner has recognized cirrhosis, they'll also examine for typical side effects. Portal hypertension is the most prevalent side effect and comes with its own set of problems, each requiring specific therapies.

You might need:

- A minor procedure to plug a bleeding vein.
- Blood transfusion to replace blood cell count.
- Kidney dialysis.

- Oxygen therapy.
- Paracentesis and antibiotics for ascites.
- Laxatives to absorb and eliminate toxins from your GI tract

Liver cancer

Primary liver cancer (hepatocellular carcinoma) is another possible consequence of cirrhosis. Not everyone with cirrhosis develops liver cancer, although most people who do develop liver cancer have cirrhosis. If you acquire cancer with cirrhosis, your provider might treat it with cancer medicines

like radiation or chemotherapy. Or they could determine that the best solution is a total liver transplant.

Liver transplantation

Healthcare providers recommend liver transplantation when they feel that your health will continue to decrease without one. This might be the case if you are in active liver failure, have liver cancer and/or you aren't responding to treatment for your liver condition. If you satisfy the conditions for a liver transplant, you'll join a nationwide waiting list to receive one. Your condition will determine your spot on the list.

Prevention

You might be able to prevent liver disease from advancing to cirrhosis by intervening earlier in the process. This depends on whether you're aware of it and whether there are things you can take to prevent it. Many people don't have symptoms in the early stages, but a simple health checkup could help bring it to light. This could provide you the chance to make crucial changes or begin treatment.

Outlook / Prognosis

Can your liver heal from cirrhosis?

Once you have cirrhosis, your liver won't get better. But it won't necessarily grow worse. If you still have compensated cirrhosis with little to no symptoms or side effects, you may continue that way for some years. If you can stop or decrease the inflammation causing cirrhosis, it may not advance to the decompensated stage. But you'll have to continue to preserve your liver for the rest of your life.

How long is life expectancy with cirrhosis liver?

Life expectancy with cirrhosis varies widely, based on several factors, including:

- How advanced it is (adjusted or decompensated).

- What complications you may have developed.

- The availability and effectiveness of treatment.

- Your overall health or additional ailments you could have

Healthcare providers employ scoring methodologies like the Child-Turcotte-Pugh (CTP) system and the Model for End-Stage Liver Disease (MELD) to anticipate your prognosis and establish your spot on the liver transplant waiting list. These ratings are based on your liver function test results and whether you have complications like ascites or hepatic encephalopathy, which would suggest decompensated cirrhosis.

Life expectancy in the early stages of compensated cirrhosis may be as high as 15 years; however, as portal hypertension develops, this decrease mostly owing to the risk of internal bleeding it can induce. The average life expectancy for decompensated cirrhosis is seven years. Severe untreatable diseases and other consequences can accelerate up that timescale. Some people have minimum two years.

How can I take care of myself while living with cirrhosis of the liver?

You can help extend the life of your liver by:

- Eating nutritious, complete meals and lean protein.
- Avoiding alcohol, tobacco and over-the-counter medications as much as possible.
- Taking drugs just as advised and discussing any prescriptions with your practitioner.
- Keeping up with basic healthcare appointments and screenings for issues.

Cirrhosis of the liver occurs in different people for different reasons. While it's typically associated with persistent alcohol use, you can also get it from problems that you're unaware of or that are beyond your control. Many people have no indication their livers are deteriorating until they develop signs of decompensated cirrhosis. Cirrhosis is a serious wake-up call once discovered.

Many liver illnesses respond to lifestyle changes and drugs. Even if you have permanent scarring, you can stop the growth of liver disease if you can stop the damage. While some cases are more complex than others, you and your provider can work out a treatment plan that will give you the best possible prognosis. If you're on the liver transplant waiting list, a transplant could save your life.

Chapter 5

Liver failure

Liver failure begins when your liver can no longer operate appropriately for your body's demands. This is also called "decompensated cirrhosis" - your body can no longer make up for the losses. As liver processes begin to break down, you'll begin to feel the impacts throughout your body. Chronic liver failure is a progressive process, but it is eventually fatal without a liver transplant. You need a liver to live.

How frequent is liver disease?

Approximately 1.8% of U.S. adults (4.5 million adults) suffer liver disease. It causes roughly 57,000 U.S. deaths a year. Globally, it causes roughly 2 million fatalities each year, or 4% of all deaths. Deaths are largely from complications of cirrhosis, with acute liver failure accounting for a minor portion. Liver disease affects men and persons assigned male at birth (AMAB) twice as often as women and those designated female at birth (AFAB).

Symptoms and Causes

In late-stage liver disease, bile doesn't move where it should. It could start to tint your skin, eyes or pee and make you itch all over.

Liver failure is a life-threatening illness that necessitates prompt medical care. Most commonly, liver failure comes gradually, over many years. It's the ultimate stage of many liver illnesses. But a rarer illness known as acute liver failure arises swiftly (in as little as 48 hours) and might be difficult to identify at first.

Liver failure arises when major sections of the liver become damaged beyond repair and the liver can't perform anymore.

There are two forms of live failure:

- **Acute:** This is when your liver stops operating within a few of days or weeks. Most persons who have this don't have any form of liver disease or condition before this event.

- **Chronic:** Damage to your liver increases over time and causes it to stop working.

Symptoms of Liver Disease and Liver Failure

The early signs of liver failure are typically similar to those of liver disorders and other ailments. Because of this, liver failure may be tricky to identify at first. Early signs include:

- Nausea
- Loss of appetite
- Fatigue
- Diarrhea

When performing properly, the liver's major job is to filter the blood entering from the digestive tract, before delivering it to the rest of the body. The liver in addition detoxifies chemicals and metabolizes medications. As it does so, the liver secretes bile which ends up back in the intestines. The liver also generates proteins needed for blood clotting and other activities.

But when liver failure worsens, the symptoms become more serious, demanding attention immediately once. These symptoms include:

- Jaundice
- Bleeding readily

- Swollen belly
- Mental confusion (known as hepatic encephalopathy)
- Sleepiness

Causes of Acute Liver Failure

The causes of acute liver failure, when the liver fails quickly, include:

- **Acetaminophen overdose:** Large doses can harm your liver or lead to failure.
- Viruses including hepatitis A, B, and E, the Epstein-Barr virus, cytomegalovirus, and herpes
- Simplex virus can also lead to liver damage or cirrhosis.
- Reactions to various prescription and natural medications: Some harm cells in your liver. Others disrupt the duct system that carries bile through it.
- **Eating deadly wild mushrooms:** A species called Amanita phalloides, popularly known as death cap, has toxins that destroy liver cells and lead to liver failure within a couple of days.
- **Autoimmune hepatitis:** As with viral hepatitis, this condition, in which your body assaults your liver, can lead to abrupt liver failure.

- **Wilson's disease:** This genetic disorder hinders your body from eliminating copper. It builds up in, and harms, your liver.
- **Acute fatty liver of pregnancy:** In this rare illness, extra fat builds on your liver and harms it.
- **Septic shock:** This overwhelming illness in your body might damage your liver or cause it to cease working.
- **Budd Chiari syndrome:** This rare condition narrows and clogs the blood vessels in your liver.
- **Industrial toxins:** Many chemicals, including carbon tetrachloride, a cleanser and degreaser, can damage your liver.

Causes of Chronic Liver Failure

- **Hepatitis B:** It makes your liver expand and hinders it from working the way it should.
- **Hepatitis C:** If you have it long-term, it can progress to cirrhosis
- **Long-term alcohol consumption:** It also contributes to cirrhosis.

- **Hemochromatosis:** This genetic illness causes your body to absorb and accumulate too much iron which can build up in the liver and cause cirrhosis

Other conditions that might lead to liver failure include:

- **Hepatitis A:** Contact with food or water infected with the hepatitis A virus, or with someone who's infected with virus, can cause liver inflammation. This variety normally goes away on its own.

- **Autoimmune hepatitis:** In this form, your body's immune system, not a virus, attacks your liver and causes inflammation.

- **Cirrhosis:** Things like drinking alcohol for many years or having hepatitis scar your liver might make it hard or impossible for your liver to perform.

- **Primary sclerosing cholangitis:** This disease steadily affects your bile ducts. It mostly affects young guys.

- **Oxalosis**: This is when the kidneys can't get rid of calcium oxalate crystals through the urine and it spreads to other parts of the body.

- **Wilson's disease:** People with this rare genetic condition store too much copper in their brain and liver.

- **Alpha-1 antitrypsin deficiency:** This genetic disorder can lead to lung or liver illness.

- **Liver cancer:** People with long-term hepatitis B or hepatitis C typically get this.

- **Liver adenoma:** In this case benign liver tumors are on an otherwise healthy liver. This typically affects women between ages 20 and 44.

- **Fatty liver disease:** Extra fat cells can develop up on your liver. Nonalcoholic fatty liver disease commonly affects patients who are overweight, obese, or have high cholesterol. Alcohol-related fatty liver disease affects people who are heavy drinkers.

- **Alcoholic hepatitis:** Liver inflammation that occurs from heavy or long-term drinking.

- **Alagille syndrome:** A genetic condition that results in fewer bile ducts than normal in the liver.

- **Primary biliary cholangitis (PBC):** Over time, this condition kills your small bile ducts. You could still hear it named by its original name, primary biliary cirrhosis.

- **Galactosemia:** People with this disorder can't process galactose, a sugar contained in many meals. It can cause liver damage.

- **Lysosomal acid lipase deficiency (LAL-D):** With this hereditary disorder, you can't create an enzyme called lysosomal acid lipase (LAL), which helps your body break down fats and cholesterol in your cells. As a result, fats linger in your liver and cause harm.

Liver Disease Progression

Stage 1: **Inflammation:** In the early stages, the liver might be inflamed and could be tender. Or it may not bother you at all.

Stage 2: **Fibrosis/scarring:** If you don't address the inflammation, it will create scarring. As scar tissue grows up in your liver, it blocks blood flow, which hinders the healthy components from doing their function and makes them work harder.

Stage 3: **Cirrhosis:** The scar tissue takes control, and with less and less good tissue to do its function, your liver won't work well, or it won't work at all.

Stage 4: **End-stage liver failure/disease:** This is an umbrella phrase for various disorders, including swelling liver, internal bleeding, loss of kidney function, fluid in your belly, and lung difficulties. Only a liver transplant can be used to cure it.

Liver Disease Diagnosis and Tests

Tests and techniques used to identify liver failure and liver disease include:

Blood testing: These let your doctor know how well your liver is performing. You might get a prothrombin time test, which evaluates how long it takes your blood to clot. With acute liver failure, blood doesn't clot as rapidly as it should.

Imaging testing: These take photographs that let your doctor examine what's going on in your liver and find out what's causing the problem. They may recommend Ultrasound, Abdominal computerized tomography (CT) scanning and Magnetic resonance imaging (MRI)

Biopsy: The doctor will use a needle to take a small sample of liver tissue and look at it in the lab. A transjugular liver biopsy is a specific treatment that lets the doctor place the needle into a vein in your neck.

How Is Liver Failure Treated?

Medication: Acetylcysteine can restore acute liver failure caused by an acetaminophen overdose. But you have to take it soon. There are also medications that can counteract the effects of mushrooms or other toxins.

Supportive care: If a virus causes liver failure, a hospital can treat your symptoms while the illness runs its course. In certain circumstances, the liver will sometimes recover on its own.

Liver transplant: If your liver failure stems from long-term damage, the initial step may be to try to save whatever part of your liver still functional. If it fails, you'll require a liver transplant. Fortunately, this surgery is often successful.

Complications of Liver Failure

Doctors will attempt to prevent problems, which include:

Cerebral edema: Fluid accumulation is a concern with liver failure. In addition to your stomach, it can also pool in your brain and cause to high blood pressure there.

Blood clotting disorders: Your liver plays a key part in helping your blood clot. When it can't accomplish its job, you're at risk of bleeding too freely.

Infections, such pneumonia and UTIs. End-stage liver illness can make you more vulnerable to catch infections.

Kidney failure: Liver failure can affect the way your kidneys perform and ultimately to failure.

How Can Liver Failure Be Prevented?

The greatest strategy to prevent liver failure is to decrease your risk of having cirrhosis or hepatitis.

Here are some strategies to help prevent these conditions:

1. Get a hepatitis vaccine or an immunoglobulin shot to prevent hepatitis A and B.
2. Eat a proper diet from all of the food groups.
3. Maintain a healthy weight.
4. Do not drink alcohol in excess. stay away from alcohol when you are taking acetaminophen.

5. Practice proper hygiene since germs are usually distributed by hands; make sure to wash your hands

completely after you use the bathroom. Also, wash your hands before touching any food

6. Don't share any personal toiletry goods, including toothbrushes and razors.

7. If you receive a tattoo or a body piercing, be sure the settings are sanitary and all equipment is aseptic (free of disease-causing germs).

8. Be mindful to utilize barrier protection (condoms) when having sex.

9. If you use illicit intravenous drugs, don't share needles with anyone.

What are the early indications and symptoms of liver disease?

In the early stages of chronic liver disease, symptoms are often absent. But occasionally it begins with a bout of acute hepatitis. For example, if you develop a viral hepatitis infection, there's an acute phase before the chronic phase comes in. You can feel a fever, stomachache or nausea for a brief period as your immune system works to defeat the infection. If it doesn't fight it, it becomes a chronic infection.

Some other types of liver disease might also begin with more severe symptoms or have occasional episodes of acute symptoms. Early indications of liver illness tend to be nonspecific. They might include:

- Upper abdominal ache.
- Nausea or loss of appetite.
- Fatigue and malaise (feeling generally tired and unwell).

What are the indications and symptoms of later-stage liver disease?

You might begin to notice additional symptoms when your liver function begins to decline. This happens in the final stages of liver disease. One of the first side effects of diminishing liver function is that bile flow slows in your biliary system. Your liver no longer makes or transmits bile adequately to your small intestine. Instead, bile begins to flow into your bloodstream. This causes certain symptoms, including:

- Jaundice (yellow tinge to the whites of your eyes and skin).
- Dark-colored pee (urine).
- Light-colored excrement (stool).
- Digestive issues, especially with lipids.
- Weight loss and muscle loss.
- Musty-smelling breath.
- Mild brain dysfunction (hepatic encephalopathy).

- Pruritus (itchy skin, but with no visible rash).

As liver disease worsens, it might alter your blood flow, hormones and nutritional status. This can manifest up in numerous ways. You may detect signs and symptoms in your skin and nails, such as

- Spoon nails.
- Terry's nails.
- Nail clubbing.
- Spider angiomas.
- Tiny red dots on your skin (petechiae).
- Small yellow pimples of fat deposits on your skin or eyelids.
- Easy bleeding and bruising.
- Red palms of your hands.

You may detect evidence of fluids leaking from your blood vessels and accumulating in your body, such as:

- Swollen abdomen (ascites).
- Swollen ankles, feet, hands and face (edema).

Liver disease symptoms in those assigned female at birth may include:

- Irregular periods (menstruation).
- Female infertility.

Liver disease symptoms in those assigned male at birth may include:
- Shrunken testicles.
- Enlarged male breast tissue.

What are the complications of end-stage liver disease?

End-stage liver disease refers to decompensated cirrhosis and liver failure, when your liver has lost the ability to regenerate and is progressively decreasing. The most serious adverse effects of end-stage liver disease are portal hypertension and primary liver cancer (hepatocellular carcinoma). Complications of these two disorders are the primary causes of

hospitalization and death in persons with cirrhosis and liver failure.

Portal hypertension

Portal hypertension arises when scarring in your liver compresses the portal vein that passes through it. High blood pressure in the portal vein causes your body to shift blood flow to other veins connected with it, which grow swollen and stretched thin. These veins might leak, rupture and bleed. Internal bleeding from these varices can be sudden, severe and life-threatening.

Additional issues, however rare, include:

Enlarged and overactive spleen (hypersplenism).

Respiratory failure (hepatopulmonary syndrome).

Kidney failure (hepatorenal syndrome).

What are the causes of liver disease?

There are approximately 100 forms of liver disease, however they fall into a handful of subgroups. Causes include:

Viral infections: Viral hepatitis infections that become chronic may cause chronic hepatitis, which includes hepatitis B and hepatitis C.

Alcohol-induced hepatitis: Heavy alcohol use can induce acute or chronic hepatitis. If it carries on long enough, it can induce cirrhosis and liver failure.

Toxic hepatitis: Chronic overexposure to contaminants, such as industrial chemicals or pharmaceuticals, can induce acute or chronic hepatitis.

Non-alcohol related fatty liver disease: Metabolic disorders associated with obesity, high blood sugar and high blood lipids can create excess fat storage in your liver, which can cause inflammation (non-alcohol related steatohepatitis).

Biliary stasis: Congenital (existing at birth) diseases that impede or stop the flow of bile via your bile ducts can cause bile to build up and harm your liver, including biliary atresia and cystic fibrosis. Non-congenital causes may include biliary stricture and gallstones.

Autoimmune disorders: Autoimmune disorders can cause persistent inflammation and scarring in your liver or your bile ducts, including autoimmune hepatitis, primary biliary cholangitis and primary sclerosing cholangitis.

Inherited metabolic disorders: Disorders that cause toxic compounds to build up in your blood — such as glycogen storage disease (GSD), Wilson disease, hemochromatosis and Gaucher disease — can cause persistent liver damage.

Cardiovascular illnesses: Conditions that influence blood flow to and from your liver — including Budd-Chiari syndrome, ischemia, vascular illnesses and right-sided heart failure — can cause persistent liver damage.

What are the risk factors for having liver disease?

You may be more likely to have liver disease if you:

1. Drink alcohol heavily.
2. Use intravenous drugs.
3. Use pain relievers like aspirin or acetaminophen
4. Have metabolic syndrome.
5. Are regularly exposed to harmful chemicals.
6. Are regularly exposed to other people's blood or body fluids.

Diagnosis and Tests

How do you test for liver disease?

A healthcare provider checking for liver illness will begin by physically examining you. They'll examine for visual clues and ask about your symptoms. They may also question about your food, lifestyle and health history. Finally, they'll utilize blood testing and imaging studies to check for liver disease. These may include:

- **Blood testing:** A panel of liver function tests can identify symptoms of liver disease, liver disease severity and liver failure. These determine liver products like liver enzymes, proteins and bilirubin levels in your blood. Blood tests may also show inflammation, specific disorders or side effects, such impaired blood clotting.

- **Imaging testing:**An abdominal ultrasound, CT scan (computed tomography scan) or MRI (magnetic resonance imaging) can indicate the size, shape and texture of your liver. This can reveal inflammation and edema, growths and fibrosis.
- **Elastography:** A unique form of imaging test called elastography employs ultrasound or MRI technologies to detect the level of stiffness or fibrosis in your liver.
- **Endoscopy:**If your physician needs to view into your biliary tract, they might need to employ a sort of endoscopic imaging. Endoscopy includes passing a tiny camera (endoscope) through your upper GI tract. From the endoscope, they can use EUS or ERCP to determine your bile ducts.

- **Nuclear medicine imaging:** A nuclear liver and spleen scan uses a gamma camera to detect a (harmless) radioactive tracer material that's injected into your body. How your liver absorbs the tracer will reveal the parts that aren't working regularly.

- **Liver biopsy:** A liver biopsy is a minor surgery to extract a small tissue sample from your liver to evaluate in a lab. A healthcare provider usually obtain the sample through a hollow needle. You could need a liver biopsy to screen for malignancy or confirm cirrhosis and help pinpoint the reason.

Chapter 6

What is alcoholic liver disease?

Alcoholic liver damage is frequent, but can be prevented. There are 3 types. Many heavy drinkers pass through these 3 types over time:

Fatty liver: Fatty liver is the accumulation of fat inside the liver cells. It leads to an enlarged liver. It's the most prevalent alcohol-induced liver issue.

Alcoholic hepatitis: Alcoholic hepatitis can be described an acute inflammation of the liver. There occurs death of liver cells, often followed by lifelong scarring.

Alcoholic cirrhosis: Alcoholic cirrhosis is the breakdown of normal liver tissue. It leaves scar tissue in place of the functional liver tissue.

The liver is a big organ that sits up under the ribs on the right side of the belly (abdomen). The liver:

- Helps filter waste from the body
- Makes bile to help digest food
- Stores sugar that the body uses for energy
- Makes proteins that act in many areas in the body, for example, proteins that induce blood to clot

What causes alcoholic liver disease?

Alcoholic liver disease is caused by heavy intake of alcohol. The liver's responsibility is to break down alcohol. If you drink more than it can process, it can become gravely injured.

Fatty liver can happen in anyone who consumes alcohol a lot. Alcoholic hepatitis and alcoholic cirrhosis are associated to the long-term alcohol abuse seen in alcoholics.

Healthcare providers don't know why some people who drink alcohol suffer liver disease while others do not. Research implies there may be a genetic relationship, but this is not yet obvious.

What are the signs of alcoholic liver disease?

The effects of alcohol on the liver are based on how much and how long you have been drinking alcohol. Fatty liver often creates no symptoms.

Below are the most common symptoms and signs:

- Build-up of fat inside the liver cells enlarges the liver, producing upper abdominal (belly) discomfort on the right side
- Tiredness and weakness

- Weight loss

- Alcoholic hepatitis
- Pain over the liver
- Fever
- Weakness
- Nausea and vomiting
- Appetite loss
- Yellowing of the skin and eyes (jaundice)

Alcoholic cirrhosis, all of the signs of alcoholic hepatitis are:

- Portal hypertension (High resistance to blood flow through the liver)
- Enlarged spleen
- Poor nutrition
- Bleeding in the intestines
- Ascites (fluid build-up in the belly)
- Kidney failure
- Confusion

Liver cancer

The signs of alcoholic liver damage may look like other health concerns. Always see a doctor for a diagnosis.

How is alcoholic liver disease diagnosed?

Your healthcare professional will do a full health history and physical assessment. Other tests used to determine alcohol-induced liver damage may include:

Blood testing, including liver function tests, which show if the liver is performing the way it should.

Liver biopsy: This includes extracting tiny tissue samples from the liver with a needle or during surgery. These samples are evaluated under a microscope to find out the type of liver illness.

Ultrasound: This test employs high frequency sound waves to build an image of the organs.

CT scan: This imaging test utilizes X-rays and a computer to produce images (commonly termed slices) of the body. A CT scan displays detailed images of any area of the body, including the bones, muscles, fat, and organs. CT scans are more comprehensive than conventional X-rays.

MRI: MRI employs a magnetic field, radio frequency pulses, and a computer to produce detailed photographs of inside body components. Sometimes injecting dye into a vein is used to make photographs of body sections. The dye assist to show the liver and other organs in the abdomen (belly).

Alcoholic Liver Disease Treatment

The goal of treatment is to restore some or all normal functionality to the liver. This may involve an alcohol treatment program, food adjustments, or other techniques.

What are the complications of alcoholic liver disease?

About 30% of persons with alcoholic liver damage have hepatitis C virus. Others have hepatitis B virus. Your provider will test you for both and treat you if necessary. People with alcoholic liver disease are also at greater risk for liver cancer.

Those with cirrhosis often have kidney difficulties, intestinal bleeding, fluid in the belly, disorientation, liver cancer, and serious infections.

Facts about alcoholic liver diseases

Alcoholic liver damage is a prevalent, but preventable, condition.

Alcoholic liver disease is caused by heavy intake of alcohol. The liver breaks down alcohol. If you drink more than it can digest, it can get badly injured.

The effects of alcohol on the liver depend on how much and how long you have been taking alcohol.

The most critical element of rehab is to fully stop consuming alcohol. Sometimes food adjustments are indicated, too.

- The liver is typically able to repair some of the damage caused by alcohol so that you can live a normal life. In some circumstances, liver transplant may be considered. But you must complete a recovery program and go through alcohol detoxification before can be an option.

Chapter 7

What Is Palmar Erythema?

Palmar erythema is a skin ailment that makes the palms of your hands turn red. It might be genetic but can also be the outcome of a range of health issues. It's also pretty prevalent throughout pregnancy.

Palmar erythema is sometimes known as liver palms, red palms, or Lane's illness.

Symptoms of Palmar Erythema

Here are some techniques to identify if the redness on your palms is palmar erythema:

- It's symmetrical — that is, the redness emerges on both palms.
- The redness is blanchable, meaning if you press on it, it fades away.
- Your palms feel somewhat heated.
- It's not painful and nor itchy.

The redness usually affects the lower half of your palm but may extend to your fingers. In certain situations, it may extend over the fingertips to the nail beds. If there is redness on the soles of your feet, it can be referred to as plantar erythema.

What Causes the Redness?

Your palms have grown red because of dilated capillaries, which are the smallest blood vessels in your body. How red your palms get seems to vary with how bad the underlying condition is. Some studies believe this has to do with higher hormone levels.

Primary Palmar Erythema

Primary palmar erythema might be genetic or caused by pregnancy.

Pregnancy is a prevalent cause of palmar erythema. It's estimated that it happens in roughly two-thirds of lighter-skinned pregnant women and up to one-third of darker-skinned pregnant women. This may happen because of changes to your blood arteries connected to an increase in estrogen production during pregnancy.

Many of the changes to your blood vessels in pregnancy are transient and subside soon after you give birth.

Palmar erythema can also be inherited, however it is a relatively unusual disorder. The redness of the palms might emerge at birth or later in life and continue from then on. This may happen to at least two members of the family, but occasional isolated cases have also been reported.

There are no indicators of inflammation, allergic response, or other health issues that have been connected to palmar erythema.

In certain circumstances, palmar erythema may be idiopathic. This signifies that there's no recognized reason and you have no other connected health concerns.

Secondary Palmar Erythema

Secondary palmar erythema might be the result of an underlying medical condition, medicine, or environmental sources. There is a broad variety of probable underlying diseases that can cause it.

Liver illness: Palmar erythema is connected with numerous forms of liver disorders. About 23% of people with liver cirrhosis have palmar erythema.

Other liver disorders connected to palmar erythema include rare liver diseases including Wilson Disease, an inherited disorder in which excessive amounts of copper build up in your body, and hereditary hemochromatosis, in which your body absorbs too much iron from the food you eat.

Babies and young toddlers with liver disease are less likely to have palmar erythema than teenagers and adults.

Autoimmune disorders: Rheumatoid arthritis is a common autoimmune and inflammatory illness that causes painful swelling in the joints and other regions of the body.

In a study of 152 patients with rheumatoid arthritis, 61% were found to have palmar erythema. Another study compared patients with rheumatoid arthritis with those who had other internal disorders.

Palmar erythema was substantially higher in patients with rheumatoid arthritis.

Other conditions that have been related with palmar erythema include:

Diabete: People with diabetes likely to suffer skin infections, and their wounds also heal slowly. An estimated 4.1% of persons with Type 1 and Type 2 diabetes mellitus develop palmar erythema.

Thyroid illness: Palmar erythema affects up to 18% of persons with thyrotoxicosis, which is when you have too much thyroid hormones in your blood.

Brain tumors: In a study of 107 persons with brain tumors, 25% were found to have palmar erythema. The severity of the redness depends on the type of tumor and its growth.

HIV: There has been one recorded incidence of palmar erythema connected to HIV.

Medications: Some drugs may produce palmar erythema. For example, suppose you take topiramate for treatment of paranoid schizophrenia. In a rare incidence, a pregnant lady administered albuterol to prevent premature labor had palmar erythema.

Other medicines that may be connected to palmar erythema include amiodarone, gemfibrozil, and cholestyramine.

Environmental causes: Smoking, drunkenness, and mercury exposure are among environmental causes of palmar erythema.

There are a few other probable disorders that researchers suggest may be connected with palmar erythema. These include:

Skin conditions: A recent incidence of palmar erythema in a three-year-old kid with no other symptoms had doctors baffled until they heard that he had been using hand sanitizer every 20 to 30 minutes throughout the day. They determined that it had an atypical presentation of contact dermatitis.

COVID-19: Skin rashes have emerged in some patients with COVID-19. In one case of a lady who tested positive for Covid-19, palmar erythema was the only symptom. She didn't have other usual COVID-19 symptoms, nor did she have other health issues related to palmar erythema.

How Is Palmar Erythema Treated?

There's no conventional treatment for palmar erythema. If you have an underlying condition causing the palmar erythema, your doctor will seek to address it. If the cause is tied to a medicine, it's suggested to discontinue it or move to a different class of drug.

What is fatty liver disease?

Fatty liver disease (steatosis) is a frequent disorder caused by having too much fats build up in your liver. A healthy liver has a little amount of fat. It becomes a concern when fat reaches 5% to 10% of your liver's weight.

Why is fatty liver disease bad?

In most cases, fatty liver disease doesn't cause any major difficulties or hinder your liver from functioning regularly. But for 7% to 30% of patients with the illness, fatty liver disease gets worse with time. It evolves via three stages:

Your liver becomes swollen (inflamed), which damages its tissue. This stage is called steatohepatitis.

Scar tissue forms where your liver is damaged. This process is termed fibrosis.

Extensive scar tissue replaces healthy tissue. At this time, you have cirrhosis of the liver.

What are the kinds of fatty liver disease?

There are two major kinds of fatty liver disease:

Alcohol-induced fatty liver disease

Alcohol-induced fatty liver disease is caused by frequent alcohol consumption. About 5% of people in the U.S. suffer this form of liver disease.

Non-alcohol related fatty liver disease

Non-alcohol related fatty liver disease (NAFLD) isn't related to alcohol usage. The disorder affects one in three adults and one in 10
children in the United States. Researchers haven't determined the exact etiology of non-alcohol related fatty liver disease. Several factors, including as obesity and diabetes, can raise your risk.

Symptoms and Causes

You have an increased probability of developing fatty liver disease if you:

- Are of Hispanic or Asian origin.
- Have completed menopause (your periods have ended).
- Have obesity with a significant level of belly fat.
- Have high blood pressure, diabetes or high cholesterol.
- Have obstructive sleep apnea (a clogged airway that causes breathing to stop and start during sleep)

What causes fatty liver disease?

Some people obtain fatty liver disease without having any pre-existing problems. But these risk factors make you more likely to develop it:

- Having overweight/obesity.

- Having Type 2 diabetes or insulin resistance.

- Having metabolic syndrome (insulin resistance, high blood pressure, high cholesterol and high triglyceride levels).

- Taking some prescription medications, such as amiodarone , diltiazem , tamoxifen or steroids.

What are the signs of fatty liver disease?

People with fatty liver disease frequently have no symptoms until the disease advances to cirrhosis of the liver. If you do have symptoms, they may include:

- Abdominal pain or a sense of fullness in the upper right side of the abdomen (belly).

- Nausea, loss of appetite or weight loss.

- Yellowish complexion and whites of the eyes (jaundice).

- Swollen abdomen and legs (edema).

- Extreme fatigue or mental disorientation.

- Weakness.

How is fatty liver disease treated?

There's no medication especially for fatty liver disease. Instead, clinicians focus on helping you manage conditions that contribute to the disorder. They also propose making lifestyle adjustments that can dramatically enhance your health. Treatment includes:

- Avoiding booze.
- Losing weight.
- Taking drugs to treat diabetes, cholesterol and triglycerides (fat in the blood).
- Taking vitamin E plus thiazolidinediones (drugs used to treat diabetes) in specified cases .

Prevention

The greatest method to avoid fatty liver disease is to perform the activities that preserve general health:

- Stay at a healthy weight. If you have overweight/obesity, lose weight gradually.
- Exercise regularly.
- Limit your alcohol consumption.
- Take drugs as prescribed.

Can fatty liver disease be reversed?

The liver has an extraordinary ability to mend itself. If you avoid alcohol or lose weight, it's feasible to minimize liver fat and inflammation and reverse early liver damage.

Will fatty liver disease kill you?

Fatty liver disease doesn't pose serious difficulties for most people. However, it can turn into a more serious condition if it progresses into cirrhosis of the liver. Untreated liver cirrhosis eventually leads to liver failure or cancer. You cannot survive or live without your liver.

What is a decent fatty liver diet?

Maintain a balanced diet to lose weight gradually but steadily. Rapid weight loss can potentially make fatty liver disease worse. Doctors generally advocate the Mediterranean diet, which is abundant in vegetables, fruits and beneficial fats. Ask your doctor or nutritionist for assistance on healthy weight loss techniques.

What are the therapies for fatty liver disease?

Doctors prescribe weight loss for nonalcoholic fatty liver. Weight loss can reduce fat in the liver, inflammation, and fibrosis. If your doctor thinks that a particular medicine is the cause of your NAFLD, you should avoid taking that medicine. But check with your doctor before quitting the medicine.

You may need to get off the prescription gradually, and you might need to switch to another medicine instead.

There are no drugs that have been authorized to treat NAFLD. Trials are studying if a certain diabetes drug or Vitamin E will assist, but additional trials are needed.

The most crucial element of treating alcohol-related fatty liver disease is to stop drinking alcohol. If you need assistance, you should speak with a therapist or enroll in an alcohol rehabilitation program. There are also drugs that can help, either by lowering your cravings or making you feel nauseous if you consume alcohol.

Both alcoholic fatty liver disease and one type of nonalcoholic fatty liver disease (nonalcoholic steatohepatitis) can progress to cirrhosis. Doctors can address the health problems produced by cirrhosis with drugs, surgeries, and other medical procedures. If the cirrhosis advances to liver failure, you may need a liver transplant.

What are some lifestyle modifications that can help with fatty liver disease?

If you have any of the kinds of fatty liver disease, there are several lifestyle adjustments that can help:

- Eat a balanced diet, reducing sodium and sugar, and eating lots of fruits, veggies, and whole grains
- Get immunizations for hepatitis A and B, the flu and pneumococcal illness. If you develop hepatitis A or B coupled with fatty liver, it is more likely to lead to liver failure. People with chronic liver illness are more likely to catch infections, thus the other two immunizations are equally crucial.
- Get regular exercise, which can help you lose weight and reduce fat in the liver.
- Talk with your doctor before using dietary supplements, such as vitamins, or any complementary or alternative treatments or medical practices. Some herbal remedies can damage your liver.

AST (SGOT)

An AST blood test examines levels of aspartate aminotransferase (AST) and helps indicate liver function. Too much of this enzyme can suggest an issue, such as liver damage.

Aspartate aminotransferase (AST) is an enzyme primarily present in the liver. AST is also present in other regions of the body such as kidney,heart and muscles.

Another term for the AST enzyme is serum glutamic-oxaloacetic transaminase (SGOT).

Most persons have low amounts of the AST enzyme. Damage to liver cells can trigger the release of additional AST into the blood however, leading to increased levels of the enzyme.

Why is the AST test performed?

Doctors typically use the AST blood test to screen for and assess liver disorders, frequently alongside other liver testing. The AST protein occurs mostly in the liver and heart. With liver disease, AST can leak from the liver into the circulation. When this happens, AST levels in the blood will be greater than normal.

AST also occurs in the brain, heart, kidneys, and muscles. If there is damage in any of these regions, AST levels may also increase.

People may have an AST test for screening, diagnostic, or monitoring purposes. A doctor may suggest this test if a person:

Possesses risk factors for liver disease, such as family history, obesity, or diabetes

Shows symptoms of a liver disease, such as jaundice, fatigue, or unexplained weight loss
is getting therapy for a liver problem, as an AST blood test can help reveal how effectively medication is working.

What level of AST is concerning?

After taking a blood test, doctors will describe AST values as normal, high, or low. Laboratories may utilize different testing procedures for examining samples, hence normal ranges can vary across each laboratory. The ranges can also vary dependent on age, sex, weight, and race, yet can still be considered normal.

The measurements for AST levels are commonly in units per liter (U/L) or international units per liter (IU/L). On a test result, the laboratory will normally mention their specific reference range.

People will need to look at this reference range and discuss with their doctor what their test findings indicate for them.

What level of AST is dangerous?

In adults, >1,000 U/L is considered a very high level and may be a symptom of liver damage or hepatitis.

The results of an AST blood test can help indicate the health of the liver.

If AST levels are high, it may also be an indication of:

- Chronic hepatitis
- Damage from alcohol
- Cholestasis, a reduction in bile flow
- Heart, kidney, bone, or muscular injury
- Liver cancers
- Liver scarring, known as liver cirrhosis
- Very high AST levels are frequently a symptom of increasing liver damage, often owing to severe hepatitis.

Low AST levels may indicate:
- Vitamin B6 deficiency
- Renal disease
- Liver disease
- Cirrhosis
- Cancer
- Autoimmune conditions
- Genetic conditions

What does high AST and ALT indicate?

Just having elevated AST with no other symptoms does not always indicate a health problem. For this reason, healthcare providers may additionally test levels of alanine aminotransferase (ALT), another liver enzyme.

ALT levels exist in higher amounts in the liver. Looking at both ALT and AST values might offer a doctor a clearer understanding of overall liver function and health.

If ALT levels are normal but AST levels are high, it could signal a health condition outside of the liver, or it may be a symptom of alcohol-induced liver damage. However, if both AST and ALT values are high, it may suggest an issue with a person's liver.

How is the AST test done?

The AST blood test is basic and identical to any other blood test. A healthcare professional may consider taking the following steps:

Sit the individual down and place a stretchy band around the upper arm to enhance blood flow to that area.

Disinfect the spot of the blood draw with an antibacterial wipe.

Inject a needle into a vein in the arm to draw a blood sample, which may cause people to experience a minor prick or pain.

Remove the needle once they have extracted enough blood.

Transmit the blood sample to a laboratory for examination.

An AST blood test will normally only take a few minutes in total.

In rare situations, patients may be able to take an AST test at home. Using an at-home test kit, consumers will collect a blood sample from their fingertips and send the sample to a laboratory. People may receive AST blood test results by the mail, an app, or an online method.

How to prepare for an AST test?

People may need to fast for several hours if they are having a combination of liver enzyme testing.

If people are merely having an AST blood test, they may not need to fast or prepare in any way.

People will need to let their doctor know if they are taking any drugs or supplements, as some may interact with liver enzyme levels.

As a healthcare expert will be collecting blood from the arm, it may be useful to wear short sleeves throughout the test.

What are the hazards of the AST test?

As with any blood test, an AST blood test has very few risks. It is rare to encounter any significant adverse effects, but patients may have some slight bruising or soreness in the area near the site of the blood draw.

A healthcare expert will place a Band-Aid or bandage on the arm to halt any bleeding.

People may wish to have something to eat following the test, particularly if they were fasting previously. It is safe for people to drive and continue their routine activities after an AST blood test unless they notice any unusual symptoms.

CONCLUSION

At one time, practically every liver ailment was fatal. Those days are behind us, better testing, treatments, and advanced knowledge have made many liver illnesses curable or reversible. But liver disease remains a severe killer and, wherever possible, prevention is always the best medicine.

It comes down to common sense, controlling diabetes, weight, and blood pressure, eating a good diet, and exercising. Moderating alcohol is crucial. Current recommendations advocate limiting alcohol to two drinks per day for males and one per day for women, but I can see that recommendation becoming one drink per day for everyone shortly.

Every adult should get an annual liver function blood test, which is especially critical if you have other risk factors. Be sure your primary care physician orders a liver panel during your annual test and be honest with your healthcare provider. No one will judge you. We help you best when we know the complete story.

It's vital to know that your liver can mend and regenerate. As the liver heals, good changes occur throughout the body. The changes can include improvements in how your digestive system performs how your skin looks and feels better mental clarity, and higher energy levels.

Your liver can recover and renew. Liver tissue can come back after it undergoes harm or a doctor removes it. This is because the liver can increase existing liver cells. New liver cells then develop and replicate in the injury or removal location.

Quitting alcohol, if feasible, is a vital step that can help your liver repair. The first week away from drinking might induce withdrawal symptoms such as headache, vomiting, insomnia, nausea, anxiety as your body adjusts to not having alcohol.

Healing can occur during the first several days after drinking ceases. Depending on the degree of the injuries, total healing can take weeks or months.

However, not all harm is reversible. If liver damage is substantial and has been long-term, it might not be able to reverse all of it. Your doctor will review the degree of your liver damage, and how much of it can repair, with you.

Doctors can cure many liver illnesses or manage them if you seek early therapy. However, liver disease is dangerous. Getting therapy as soon as possible will help you prevent permanent damage.

www.ingramcontent.com/pod-product-compliance
Lightning Source LLC
Chambersburg PA
CBHW062340290526
45794CB00005B/2068